ICS 01.040.11

SCM

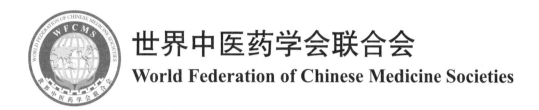

世界中医药学会联合会
World Federation of Chinese Medicine Societies

SCM 0014-2014

国际中医药学科体系类目

International Catalogue of Chinese Medicine Discipline System

2014-10-02 发布实施

中国中医药出版社

图书在版编目（CIP）数据

国际中医药学科体系类目/世界中医药学会联合会
著 . —北京：中国中医药出版社，2016.10
ISBN 978-7-5132-3424-5

Ⅰ . ①国… Ⅱ . ①世… Ⅲ . ①中国医药学—分类体系
Ⅳ . ①R2

中国版本图书馆 CIP 数据核字（2016）第 104230 号

中国中医药出版社出版
北京市朝阳区北三环东路 28 号易亨大厦 16 层
邮政编码 100013
传真 010 64405750
三河市潮河印业有限公司印刷
各地新华书店经销

*

开本 880×1230 1/16 印张 1 字数 25 千字
2016 年 10 月第 1 版 2016 年 10 月第 1 次印刷
书 号 ISBN 978-7-5132-3424-5

*

定价 18.00 元
网址 www.cptcm.com

社长热线 010 64405720
购书热线 010 64065415 010 64065413
微信服务号 zgzyycbs
书店网址 csln.net/qksd/
官方微博 http://e.weibo.com/cptcm
淘宝天猫网址 http://zgzyycbs.tmall.com

目　　次

前　言

本标准起草单位：世界中医药学会联合会秘书处。

本标准主要起草人员：李振吉、徐春波、尼古拉·罗宾逊（英国）、胡晓阳（英国）、邹建华、王晶、焦云洞、李昕雪、单梁。

本标准参与起草人员：

中国大陆（以汉语拼音为序）：曹毅、陈可冀、韩晶岩、胡义扬、黄惠勇、江丹、凯赛尔·阿不都克热木、李灿东、李济仁、梁繁荣、刘建平、刘清国、吕晓东、牛阳、乔明琦、宋柏林、唐启胜、万有、王健、肖小河、徐斌、徐宏喜、叶祖光、赵百孝、朱立国、朱晓新。中国香港：温桂荣。中国台湾：黄三德。

美国：王守东、Walter N Duráur、Li Peng、张群豪。

澳大利亚：林子强、刘炽京、张翼。

德国：Thomas Efferth。

新西兰：徐昕。

新加坡：王葆方、林钥华。

英国：樊台平。

本标准的起草程序遵守了世界中医药学会联合会发布的 SCM 0001-2009《标准制定和发布工作规范》。

本标准于 2014 年 10 月 2 日由世界中医药学会联合会第三届第六次理事会审议通过。

本标准由世界中医药学会联合会发布。版权归世界中医药学会联合会所有。

引　言

目前，全球中医药医疗、科研和高等院校尚缺乏统一适用的中医药学科分类标准。为建立统一、规范、广泛适用的中医药学科分类体系，特制定本标准，为中医医疗机构、科研院所、高等院校等开展临床、科研及教育提供学科分类的参考。

本标准以中华人民共和国国家中医药管理局《中医药重点学科建设专家委员会中医药学科建设规划指导目录》为基础，同时参考了相关国家中医药法律法规及科研、教育领域的相关文献资料。

本标准有助于保证中医药学科的系统性和完整性，推动中医药学科体系的完善。

国际中医药学科体系类目

1 范围

本标准规定了中医药学科的体系类目。

本标准适用于中医药学科建设、国际人才培养、科研以及教育指导工作。

2 术语和定义

下列术语和定义适用于本标准。

2.1 学科

相对独立的知识体系。

2.2 中医药学科体系

由与中医药相关的中医基础医学、中医临床医学、针灸推拿学、中药学、中西医结合医学、各类民族医药学以及培育学科组成的体系。

3 中医药学

3.1 中医基础医学

3.1.1 中医基础理论

3.1.2 内经学

3.1.3 伤寒学

3.1.4 金匮要略

3.1.5 温病学

3.1.6 中医各家学说

3.1.7 中医史学

3.1.8 中医文献学

3.1.9 古汉语与医古文

3.1.10 方剂学

3.1.11 中医诊断学

3.2 中医临床医学

3.2.1 中医内科学

3.2.1.1 中医心病学

3.2.1.2 中医肝胆病学

3.2.1.3 中医脾胃病学

3.2.1.4 中医肺病学

3.2.1.5 中医肾病学

3.2.1.6 中医脑病学

3.2.1.7 中医痹病学

3.2.1.8 中医内分泌病学

3.2.1.9 中医肿瘤病学

3.2.1.10 中医血液病学

3.2.2 中医外科学

3.2.2.1 中医皮肤病学

3.2.2.2 中医肛肠病学

3.2.2.3 中医疮疡病学

3.2.3　中医骨伤科学

3.2.4　中医妇科学

3.2.5　中医男科学

3.2.6　中医儿科学

3.2.7　中医眼科学

3.2.8　中医耳鼻喉科学

3.2.9　中医口腔科学

3.2.10　中医急诊学

3.2.11　中医养生学

3.2.12　中医康复学

3.2.13　中医老年医学

3.2.14　中医护理学

3.2.15　中医全科医学

3.3　**针灸推拿学**

3.3.1　针灸学

3.3.2　推拿学

3.4　**中药学**

3.4.1　中药资源学

3.4.1.1　药用植物学

3.4.1.2　药用动物学

3.4.1.3　药用矿物学

3.4.2　中药鉴定学

3.4.3　中药炮制学

3.4.4　中药药剂学

3.4.5　中药化学

3.4.6　中药分析学

3.4.7　中药药理学

3.4.8　临床中药学

3.5　**中西医结合**

3.5.1　中西医结合基础

3.5.2　中西医结合临床

3.6　**各类民族医药学**

3.6.1　各类民族医学

3.6.2　各类民族药学

3.7　**培育学科**

3.7.1　中医预防医学

3.7.2　中医传染病学

3.7.3　中医药信息学

3.7.4　中医药工程学

3.7.5　中医心理学

3.7.6　中医络病学

3.7.7　中医文化学

3.7.8　中国神志病学

参考文献

［1］中华人民共和国国家中医药管理局．中医药重点学科建设专家委员会中医药学科建设规划指导目录，2009．

［2］新加坡中医学院（Singapore College of Traditional Chinese Medicine）http：//www．singaporetcm．edu．sg/en/courses_ syllabus．php

［3］加拿大国际中医学院（International College of Traditional Chinese Medicine of Vancouver）http：//www．tcmcollege．com/index．php？option＝com_ content&view＝category&id＝3&Itemid＝54

［4］美洲中医学院（American College of Traditional Chinese Medicine）http：//www．actcm．edu/

［5］英国中医学院（UK Academy of Chinese Medicine）http：//www．ukacademyofchinesemedicine．co．uk/en_ page．php？id＝31

［6］中华人民共和国国务院学位委员会．学位授予和人才培养学科目录，2011．

［7］GB/T 13745－2009 学科分类与代码．

［8］中华人民共和国教育部学位委员会．授予博士、硕士学位和培养研究生的学科、专业目录，1997．

［9］中华人民共和国国家自然科学基金委员会．国家自然科学基金中医药学科相关申请标准，2015．

Foreword

Chief Drafting Organization: Secretariat of WFCMS.

Chief Drafters: Li Zhenji, Xu Chunbo, Nicola Robinson (UK), HU Xiaoyang (UK), Zou Jianhua, Wang Jing, Jiao Yundong, Li Xinxue, Shan Liang.

Participating Drafters:

China (mainland) (in alphabetical order): Cao Yi, Chen Keji, Han Jingyan, Hu Yiyang, Huang Huiyong, Jiang Dan, Kaisaier Abudukeremu, Li Candong, Li Jiren, Liang Fanrong, Liu Jianping, Liu Qingguo, Lv Xiaodong, Niu Yang, Qiao Mingqi, Song Bolin, Tang Qisheng, Wan You, Wang Jian, Xiao Xiaohe, Xu Bin, Xu Hongxi, Ye Zuguang, Zhao Baixiao, Zhu Liguo, Zhu Xiaoxin. China (Hong Kong): Wen Guirong. China (Taiwan): Huang Sande.

The United States: Wang Shoudong, Walter N Duráur, Li Peng, Zhang Qunhao.

Australia: Lin Ziqiang, Liu Chijing, Zhang Yi.

Germany: Thomas Efferth.

New Zealand: Xu Xin.

Singapore: Wang Baofang, Lin Yuehua.

Britain: Fan Taiping

International Catalogue of Chinese Medicine Discipline System is drafted in accordance with the rules based on the *SCM* 0001-2009 *Working Regulation for Formulation and Publication of Standard*.

The standard is reviewed and passed in the 6th session of the 3rd Board on October 2nd, 2014 of World Federation of Chinese Medicine Societies.

The Standard is issued by the World Federation of Chinese Medicine Societies. All rights reserved by the World Federation of Chinese Medicine Societies.

Introduction

At present, there is no universally and commonly acknoledged international standard for discipline cultivation of Chinese medicine medical research in institutions, universities and colleges all over the world. To establish a unified discipline classification system of Chinese medicine, and promote the standardization and applicability of discipline classification of Chinese medicine, this standard is established, providing basis for global course system construction, personnel training and scientific research of Chinese medicine.

This standard is based on *The Key Discipline Committee of Experts' Discipline Construction Planning Guidance Catalogue of Chinese Medicine* by State Administration of TCM of People's Republic of China, and at the same time refers to relevant laws and regulations in other countries.

The International Catalogue of Chinese Medicine Discipline System may guide the construction of Chinese medicine disciplines, improve the talents cultivation, ensure systematicness and integrity of Chinese medicine disciplines, and promote the perfection of Chinese medicine.

International Catalogue of Chinese Medicine Discipline System

1 Scope

The standard specifies the basic terms of the discipline system of Chinese medicine.

The standard applied the discipline construction and cultivation of talents of Chinese medicine .

2 Terms and Definitions

The following terms and definitions are applicable to this document.

2.1 Discipline

Relatively independent knowledge systems.

2.2 Chinese Medicine Discipline System

The system composed of relevant disciplines of Chinese medicine, such as basic medical science of Chinese medicine, Chinese medicine clinical medicine, acupuncture-moxibustion and tuina, Chinese materia medica, integrated Chinese and Western medicine, medicine of national ethnicities, cultivating discipline, for health organizations of Chinese medicine (medical and health institutions, research institutes, universities and colleges, etc.) providing clinical discipline classification, scientific research and education for guidance.

3 Chinese Medicine

3.1 Basic Medical Science of Chinese Medicine

3.1.1 Basic Theory of Chinese Medicine

3.1.2 Internal Classic

3.1.3 Treatise on Cold Damage Diseases

3.1.4 Synopsis of the Golden Chamber

3.1.5 Warm Diseases

3.1.6 Various Schools of Chinese Medicine

3.1.7 History of Chinese Medicine

3.1.8 Chinese Medicine Literature

3.1.9 Ancient Chinese and Medical Articles of Archaic Chinese

3.1.10 Chinese Medical Formulas

3.1.11 Diagnostics of Chinese Medicine

3.2 Chinese Clinical Medicine

3.2.1 Chinese Internal Medicine

3.2.1.1 Heart Diseases of Chinese Medicine

3.2.1.2 Liver and Gallbladder Diseases of Chinese Medicine

3.2.1.3 Spleen and Stomach Diseases of Chinese Medicine

3.2.1.4 Lung Diseases of Chinese Medicine

3.2.1.5 Kidney Diseases of Chinese Medicine

3.2.1.6 Brain Diseases of Chinese Medicine

3.2.1.7 Arthralgia Diseases of Chinese Medicine

3.2.1.8 Endocrine Diseases of Chinese Medicine

3.2.1.9 Tumor Diseases of Chinese Medicine

3.2.1.10 Blood Diseases of Chinese Medicine

3.2.2 Chinese External Medicine

3.2.2.1 Skin Diseases of Chinese Medicine

Bibliography

[1] State Administration of TCM of People's Republic of China. The expert committee of key discipline in the discipline Guidance catalogue of TCM, 2009.

[2] Singapore College of Traditional Chinese Medicine http: //www. singaporetcm. edu. sg/en/courses_ syllabus. php

[3] International College of Traditional Chinese Medicine of Vancouver http: //www. tcmcollege. com/index. php? option=com_ content&view=category&id=3&Itemid=54

[4] American College of Traditional Chinese Medicinehttp: //www. actcm. edu/

[5] UK Academy of Chinese Medicine http: //www. ukacademyofchinesemedicine. co. uk/en_ page. php? id=31

[6] *GB/T 13745-2009 Discipline Classification and Code.*

[7] The School Committee of The State Council of People's Republic of China. The discipline catalogue about granting Degree and cultivating talent, 2011.

[8] The school committee of the ministry of education of People's Republic of China. The disciplines and specialties catalogue of granting doctor, master's degree and cultivating postgraduate, 1997.

[9] The fund committee of national natural science of People's Republic of China. The related application standards about discipline of TCM in national natural science fund, 2015.